I0436934

PERMANENT WEIGHT LOSS
After Bariactric Surgery

Not a Magic Pill

PATSY WINZEY

Bloomington, IN  Milton Keynes, UK

authorHOUSE®

AuthorHouse™
1663 Liberty Drive, Suite 200
Bloomington, IN 47403
www.authorhouse.com
Phone: 1-800-839-8640

AuthorHouse™ UK Ltd.
500 Avebury Boulevard
Central Milton Keynes, MK9 2BE
www.authorhouse.co.uk
Phone: 08001974150

© 2007 Patsy Winzey. All rights reserved.

No part of this book may be reproduced, stored in a retrieval system, or
transmitted by any means without the written permission of the author.

First published by AuthorHouse   5/30/2007

ISBN: 978-1-4259-9212-5 (sc)

Library of Congress Control Number: 2007900703

Printed in the United States of America
Bloomington, Indiana

This book is printed on acid-free paper.

This is dedicated to my daughter,
who made me realize I had nothing to be ashamed of,
my son
the computer genius whom scanned pictures, found
files I lost, and was my most
dedicated editor,
my husband
who supported the idea and acted as my "devil's

advocate"

Preface

"Permanent Weight Loss After Bariactric Surgery" addresses the pains experienced emotionally and physically when someone is overweight. It also addresses the pain and triumphs of losing weight after Bariactric Surgery. Thousands of people have already had bariactric surgery and have found that it is not the "Magic Pill" to permanent weight loss that the majority of society believes it be. In order to be considered as a candidate for the surgery you must be at least 100 pounds over weight. There are some people that are carrying so much weight that doctors will require that they lose some of it before the surgery. Isn't it ironic that you can actually weigh too much to have a surgery that will reduce how much you weigh? However, any surgery is dangerous and doctors don't want to increase the dangers of this one by having too much girth to cut through.

If you are 100 pounds or more over weight, you must revisit your past, or recent situation, for some emotional upset that was, or isn't being addressed, or see a physician to see if there is something metabolic problem that has gone undetected. I my case it was

all three, but please hear this... being 100 or more pounds over weight is

not to be taken lightly! Not only is your life being adversely affected, but you

are causing unneeded pain and worry for anyone who knows and loves you.

The first year after the surgery, the weight miraculously disappears without any effort. However, after about a year or two patients are warned that they will gain about 10 to 15 pounds. My manuscript honestly, and personally, describes what must be done to make the weight loss permanent.

It will be of interest to the thousands of people who have already had bariactric surgery, and to the thousands that will have the surgery in the future. It will also give some insight to friends and relatives of someone with a weight problem. You may think that "they are eating themselves to death," but they are dealing with much more than the food you see them putting in their mouth's.

The following pages can also be an aide to those who have had the surgery and never reached their goal weight. As long as obesity exists in this world, bariactric surgery will exist also, and my manuscript will be of assistance. It may be of help to anyone who is struggling with their weight and would like lose it without the surgery. It encourages soul searching, and with any problem of weight control, unless there is a detectable physical reason, obesity is a problem hiding in the soul.

Living the busy lives that we all do it is a "quick read" and tells my story of lifelong yo-yo dieting, my decision to have the surgery, recovery from the surgery, and the new life I am living as a result of my decision to have the procedure done. I will discuss the ups and downs, and the pains and triumphs. I have enclosed before and after photos and the secret to making the success of this surgery permanent. My story is not told chronologically and may seem to jump time periods at times, but I am discussing the "feelings" discovered with certain events in my life. "Hang with me" and the point that I am trying to make will be made.

I hope reading my experience will help you lose the weight you have regained if you have already had the surgery. I hope it encourages you to do your homework and to make an informed decision before having the surgery. If you have had the surgery already, I hope it will help you permanently maintain your goal weight. You must make the decision; it has to be done for your benefit and your benefit alone. The world will not change. The people you live with will not change. You can only control how you react to the life you have been given. You are the only person you can control and you must gain control of the food you eat. You must become the author of your life.

Table of Contents

Your Decision

Your decision to undergo bariactric surgery for weight loss *is your decision*, and no one else's. Weight loss is a personal decision for anyone who deals with the emotional and physical difficulties of obesity. Anyone who is obese deals with the pitfalls of belonging to a subculture that is discriminated against as any minority group. The overweight must endure having to buy clothing in separate sections of stores (if not at a store specifically designed for the "Big" or "Full-figured"), not being able to fit through turn stiles designed for "normal sized" people. They are not able to fit on certain rides at amusement parks, or some seats in any theater. They are considered unattractive by society in general, and they must deal with the sneers and comments of insensitive people. Being an emotional eater, eating your feelings, eating for comfort, eating to deal with failure, eating for reward, whatever the reason for overeating enough to cause the problem of being overweight, are motivations that must be dealt with by the over-eater. To pretend that obesity is simply a physical problem and that it is not intertwined with some type of emotional disorder is a mistake that will make permanent weight loss impossible.

If you are dealing with a weight problem that you have dealt with for years on end, you must also deal with the fact that overeating causes metabolic changes in your body that actually makes losing weight harder. Some families are genetically predisposed to obesity; another factor that must be considered when it comes to weight loss. This is a factor I had to consider. Obesity is a genetic problem I've inherited from both sides of my family. Whatever the reason that has brought you to the point of considering bariactric surgery, ***you and you alone***, must make the decision. You shouldn't allow a spouse, children, or anyone else in your life to be a factor because it will be you who will have to deal with the dangers and discomforts of surgery. You will also face stressful times when you will want to overeat and your body will not allow you to, and the feelings of failure you will deal with when you allow the stress to motivate you to find inventive ways of over riding the preventive the procedure creates to keep you from over eating. If overeating is a crutch you have been using to survive mentally, 1 would advice you analyze why you use this crutch and get rid of it by "facing your demons" to get rid of it. If you don't you will replace it with some other equally detrimental vice to fill the emotional disturbance like sex addiction, drug abuse, or alcoholism, et cetera.

I was molested, on more than one occasion, as a child and this was when my weight problem began. My nickname before these events in my life was "Teeny", I was that petite. The first incident happened when I was 6 years old and my life long battle with my weight began. The second molestation happened the same year. At my first sleep over at a friend's house. This horrible event recalls to my mind one of my most loving memories of my emotionally distant mother. I can remember her leaning down to hug me and she told me before she left me that if I got scared, no matter how late, just call and she would come to pick me up. This was a suppressed memory until I started dealing with the pain of the first molestation, which was never forgotten.

I was sitting at my sewing machine one evening, and remembered some horrible things that "my best friend" from my first grade class had done to me after we were put to bed. I don't know how molesters know that we who are molested aren't strong enough to say no at the time, but when she was done with me, I had her mother call my mom to come get me. She came to my rescue at 1 a.m., with no questions asked. I never told her what happened, but this girl became someone I never spoke to again, not even at school. My mind took over and I erased the events until my mind was old enough to handle the pain.

My first experience destroyed my trust of father figures and the second made me trust very few girls, or women of my age group. I became a "tom boy" and hung out with the guys. To this day, I am some what of a loner. So any girl, or woman, that I have allowed into "my circle" since then have really been special to me. I can say the same for any a man 15 to 20 years my senior. Even once the "band-aides" over the sores of molestation are removed, I believe the scars always remain to some extent. At the time I remembered the event I became filled with anger, rage, and hurt, but now I feel sorrow for that little girl who molested me. For her to have had the knowledge to do what she did to me, I can't imagine what was being done to her.

At the age of 12 I began a vicious cycle of dieting, exercising, gaining, and going up and down the weight scale losing and gaining 50 to 70 pounds with each cycle. At 33, when my children turned 4 and 6, I began psychiatric care to deal with the emotional scars of being molested (classical reason to begin, triggered by my maternal instinct to protect my own children). After about a year of mental work, I returned to college to finish getting a teaching credential that I had begun at age 18 and threw behind me at 20, after getting married. I was happier and had the confidence I needed to return to school.

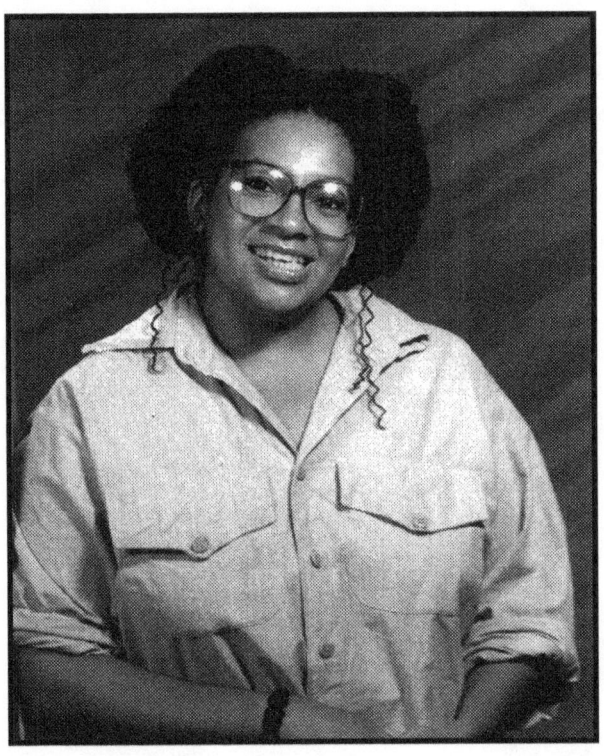

After having my daughter, my second and last child, I lost all my weight again. I was proudly wearing jeans (size 9/10) that I had worn during one of my previous weight loses. Shortly after my daughter turned 2, I packed on a whopping 80 to 90 pounds in a 9 month period and found out that I had hypothyroidism. I began taking Synthroid and will have to take it for the rest of my life.

Before I returned to school I dieted and exercised religiously to no avail. I did gain muscle, but I lost no weight. Once school started, I put my weight on hold again, promising myself that once school was finished, I would give losing weight my full attention once again.

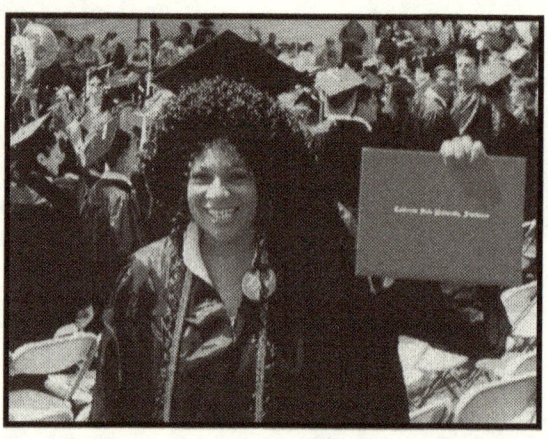

After jumping the hurdle of finishing college and getting my credential, I decided to turn attention once again to finish, and win, my lifelong marathon of weight reduction. I dieted and exercised religiously. By the time I finished school though, I weighed 315 pounds. I dieted and exercised once again for a 2 year period and lost 10 pounds. I faced the fact that the years of yo-yo dieting and the hypothyroidism had created metabolic changes in my body that made losing weight a hurdle that I was going to be unable to jump alone. I needed help.

Before I came to this realization I had tried every diet in existence. Jenny Craig was successful as long as I ate Jenny's food. Once I reached my goal weight, I regained the weight I lost. Nutri-System was also very successful for me while I ate their food. Once again, the weight returned when I returned to eating regular food. Both of these programs have a year's maintenance program that's supposed to teach you how to eat properly so the weight won't be regained. I enrolled in both of their complete programs, and in the long-run was unsuccessful. I have always been a "comfort eater". Once I left the programs, any upsetting event would put chocolate bars, ice cream, and donuts, anything I could find back into my mouth and into my stomach. Then the cycle of "I'll get back on the diet tomorrow," would begin and before I knew it, months would have past and 15 to 20 pounds would have been gained with each passing month. I tried the Hollywood Fast for 3 days diet, the Protein Power Plan, Optifast, Slimfast, Live for Life, Weight Watchers, Atkins,

Scarsdale, the Onion and Cabbage Soup Diet, and doctor prescribed appetite suppressants. You name it, I've tried it. The list is endless. The bottom line was, as long as I had the ability to overeat, *I did.*

I had a cousin who had decided to have bariactric surgery and she suggested I do some research because it is a life changing event and should not be done without considerable understanding of the procedure. I found that there are numerous web sites devoted to giving prospective candidates everything you need to know about the procedure, and the different types that are available. I was almost overwhelmed with the information available, but *I did do* my homework. I was suffering with a medical problem that I was going to need surgery to correct anyway, and my stomach was going to be opened, so I decided to get it all done at once.

The hospital that could get me scheduled for the procedure the soonest only did the "Vertical-ring Bypass Roux-en-Y Gastro-jujunostomy." In laymen's terms it is a stomach stapling or Gastric-Bypass. Every other hospital had a waiting list of at least a year, if not more. I was given a list of possible side effects that seemed endless and was quite frightening. I would also like to add at this point that gallstones are one of the listed side effects. Some bariactric doctor's remove the gall bladder as a precaution with the initial surgery to prevent having to perform another surgery in the future. Any type of rapid weight loss can cause problems with the gallbladder and with my years of gaining and losing, mine had already been removed. I pondered my options for about 6 months and when I started having problems with my knees and ankles from carrying so much weight and the beginnings of other weight related diseases. I decided the outcome "outweighed" the dangers. I was already facing high blood pressure, heart disease, cancer, and stroke because one or more of these diseases had already killed members of my maternal and paternal sides of my family. My blood pressure had begun to rise (after years of having low blood pressure), my heart would palpitate with any exertion, and my body had begun to create fatty tumors in one place after another. I had to take care of the problem in my stomach also. Time was of the essence.

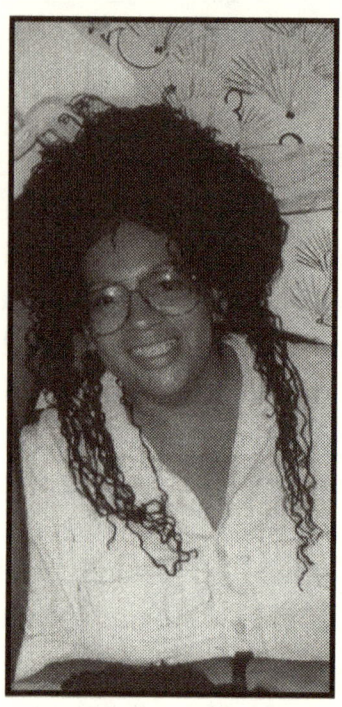

My husband's insurance would not cover any type of weight loss program or procedure, but the insurance offered through the school district where I received my first full-time teaching position did. So if bariactric surgery is something you are considering, I recommend researching what insurances that will cover the procedure first. It was disheartening for me initially to find out that my husband's insurance would not cover the procedure once I had decided to have it done. Once I found out that my insurance covered the procedure I was elated, but the initial let-down could have been avoided if my homework had been done with deeper concentration. There is a web site available that lists all participating insurance carriers that provide the surgery. Still with the joy of finding out that my insurance would cover the procedure, whoever was responsible for contracting "fair and reasonable expenses" with my insurance company at the hospital, did not do their job very well.

Sanger Hospital contacted me 4 days before the surgery to cancel the procedure. I was devastated and angry. I have been devastated and depressed before and the depression makes me very unproductive. Anger is a very good motivator for me. So I allowed the anger to take "the driver's seat." After about 20 calls I made between my insurance company and the hospital, I found out that 2 of the 20 people covered by my insurance plan had undergone the surgery. The insurance paid the hospital $1,500 for a surgery that cost over $25,000. "Off the record," someone at my insurance company told me that it was illegal for the hospital to cancel the surgery under these circumstances. Sanger is a little town on the outskirts of Fresno, California. It was a 2 hour drive, but my husband and I made the trip to talk to the hospital administrator. I told him what I knew and threatened to sue if the surgery did not proceed as planned. I had made arrangements for a long-term substitute at work and had already paid for the train ticket to get my sister to my house, and my sister had made arrangements for her responsibilities to be taken care of in her 4 week planned absence from my mother's home. Worse yet, it had taken me 6 months to mentally prepare myself and I had other health problems that were to be taken care of with this surgery.

Facing the reality of his situation the hospital administrator went ahead and re-ordered the previously cancelled surgery, the pre-op testing, and had my blood drawn after our conversation and the surgery proceeded as scheduled. (By the way, because of this mistake, Sanger General Hospital no longer exists.)

In November 2000, I had the surgery. My husband and family supported me, but it was *my* decision and *my* decision alone. I would also have to give my greatest thanks to my youngest sister, Trinity, who came and took over delegating chores, and running my household while I recovered. She had not gotten her driver's license yet. She had gotten her permit, but had never gotten her license. She mustered up the courage to do so for me when she arrived, so she would be able to take my children to and from school. We knew my husband would be spending the majority of his time with me at the hospital. I really don't think I could have let go of my responsibilities if I were not sure they would have been taken care of in my absence. She gave me the "peace of mind" to concentrate on myself.

Still, I cannot express enough that ***this decision must be yours*** so if anything does go wrong, no one else will feel responsible for your ills. Bariactric surgery is a decision that should not be taken lightly. As with any surgery death is always a possibility. You should not make anyone in your life responsible for ***your*** decision. It isn't a "Magic Pill" and it is not for everyone. Do your research. Make an informed decision, and ***decide for yourself.***

The Surgery and Recovery

The day of the surgery we left in 2 cars. My husband and I led the way as my sister followed with my kids. It had really worried me before that my kids had known about the surgery for about 2 months before, but never questioned or needed to talk about it, until that morning. I guess that's just how some kids deal with frightening events, they just don't think about them until they have to. However, that morning they both were quiet and withdrawn when we got them up for school and my son finally told us that they were worried and wanted to go with me. The surgery took about 3 hours. Once my children knew mommy was still alive and was going to survive, my sister took them home. I was in the hospital for 4 days. My husband stayed the first night and left the second day. I was bored, lonely, and I was in **pain**. I could only eat a Dixie Cup size of protein gelatin every 2 hours. I wasn't really hungry because I was nauseated and in *pain*. I welcomed the shots that would just put me to sleep for 3 to 4 hours just to get rid of the discomfort. I was told by my nurse that throwing up could tear the stitches both inside and outside my body, so even with the medicine given me for the nausea, while awake, I fought throwing up a great deal of the time I was awake.

The nurse I had also started out as Dr. Jekyll and by the end of his shift became Mr. Hyde. His shift began with my admittance and ended with my discharge. He was a male nurse and I thought it was quite the novelty. He was so sweet at first. He calmed my fears and told me everything was going to be fine, but before I went home I was almost afraid he was going to smother me in my sleep! He complained when I needed anything. I was on a continual IV drip that gave me fluids beyond what I could intake under normal circumstances, and I did have to "go" a lot. He started to complain about disturbing him when I went to the restroom. I had a room mate who had undergone the procedure also and we were both instructed not to get up without assistance. We had to take 2 walks a day and he complained about that. He was grumpy and antagonistic about any assistance I needed, changing my IV bag, adjusting and changing the sheets, adjusting and checking the circulation devices on my legs (blood clots are one of the dangers of the surgery and these are a preventative). The last "straw" for me was when he tried to make me eat one of my Dixie Cup size meals with the dirty spoon from the previous meal. I refused and said, "Would you please get me a clean spoon, and what is your problem anyway!" I got no response, he just handed me a clean spoon. The hospital did have us fill out a rating questionnaire about our stay and my nurse did not get a good recommendation from me or my room mate. We documented everything Mr. Hyde had done. I was so glad to get home, at least at first.

By the time I went home the nausea had passed. I had to remain on the protein gelatin diet for 2 weeks. I could then start adding in soft foods and soups. After a month, my doctor explained that my stomach was now the size of a large fist and I could begin adding regular foods to my diet, but in very small portions. It varies with each doctor how eating and drinking is to be handled after the surgery. I was told that since my stomach was so small, I was instructed to eat small portions of very nourishing meals and not to drink liquids with my meals because the liquids would only take up needed space. The fluids would also push the food through my stomach at a rate that would affect absorption of needed nourishment. However, water is a must! I have had the habit of carrying bottled water with me everywhere I go for about the past 15 years because I am prone to bladder and kidney infections. Water helps your liver flush fat from your system. So even if the size of your new tummy will only allow you to take 7 or 8 gulps of it at a time, make drinking water a priority between meals and snacks. I was also instructed to find a good multivitamin because my body would naturally be deprived of needed vitamins and minerals just because of the nature of the procedure. On my first post-op visit I told him I was experiencing some burning in my stomach after eating and he prescribed Prilosec. (A prelude to a nightmare ahead). I was also told to stay away from acidic foods and drinks like oranges, orange juice, and ascorbic vitamin C. After almost getting the symptoms of scurvy, I added buffered vitamin C to my regimen. I was also told to concentrate on my protein intake. He said that protein was very important for the healing process of the stomach and properly balanced with carbohydrates would add to my energy level. I complained of being very tired because I was! I only got to see my surgeon twice after the procedure because the hospital closed and he was not listed in the directory. So only 2 months after this life changing surgery, I was on my own.

I became very creative figuring out my meals. Protein shakes, Weight Watcher's pre-packaged breakfast muffins, 1 egg omelets with fat-free cheese, oatmeal, and a pancake were some of my favorite meals for breakfast. **Do not skip breakfast either!** That is a mistake that a lot of dieters make, but without breaking the fast that sleeping causes, your body will go into starvation mode. You need to get "your motor running," your metabolism that is, by having breakfast. A car will not start without gasoline, yet so many people make the mistake of making their bodies run until noon without food. It just is not conducive to making a sluggish metabolism kick into gear. For lunch a half of any type of sandwich with a few fat free chips, salads with tuna (no ice burg lettuce, I've read that this lettuce was created as a filler for cow food and is hard for our bodies to digest, and I did and still do throw it up), and a variety of soups were favorite meals for lunch. One of my favorite dinners became feta with spinach and hamburger meat. I became a lover of steak, roast, meat loaf, and vegetables. A barbequed steak with a green salad was blissfully satisfying to me. I actually craved foods that were good for me! Throughout the day I would snack on fruit and protein bars. Something else that's very helpful is to make large amounts of what you cook and freeze them into small portion sizes. I get to come home for lunch, and when I can just pop something into the microwave and not have to worry about preparing something to eat, it makes sticking to my diet so much easier. This was one of the things that made Jenny Craig and Nutri-Systems a success for me at first. Having prepared foods really helps. Another helpful tip is not to eat after 6 p.m. This isn't a rule that must be carried out rigidly. For instance, don't eat after 6 during the week, but if you go out or there is a special event on the weekend, go ahead and eat socially, just don't get carried away and forget to count your calories. I started out on 1200 calories a day, but now I stick to about 16 to 1800 a day. Not eating after 6 allows you to go to bed a little hungry, and food will be the first thing you think of in the morning. You can drink as much water or unsweetened decaffeinated tea as you wish, but adhering to this adjustment will greatly increase your desire for breakfast. Breakfast will not be skipped!

Now I can eat just about anything I want to eat except Chinese food with MSG. I will still throw up if I make this mistake. I have to ask if the restaurant uses MSG before eating any Chinese food. I do eat pizza, burgers, tacos, chips and salsa, spaghetti, shrimp Alfredo, but I am 6 years from the surgery. As the years pass the adjustments become natural. They become a part of the new you. However, it does take time. Everything I put on my plate must still be eaten in small portions. This was an adjustment that did not come easy once I started eating "normal" foods again. I would just naturally put too much food on my plate. I threw away a lot of food during this time period. Old habits die hard. It took awhile to except that thin people eat thin portions.

When I returned home from the hospital, I did discover I had more mental work to do, and not just with the physical adjustments I obviously had to face with my recovering body. I have always been a perfectionist. I was a "bastard child" during a time period when it made a big difference in the social acceptance of the child. I know it is now politically correct to say illegitimate and it really doesn't make a difference anymore, but "that bastard child" is what I heard as far back as I can remember. Now it has become so accepted by society that it is joked about with sayings such as, "This is my other baby's daddy," or "Is that yo baby's Daddy?"

At the time I mistakenly thought that being perfect would make my family forgive me for being born. My grandmother refused to have anything to do with me at first. A family across the street from my grandmother's house took me in. They offered to baby sit me for my mother while she went to work. The Coleman's became my family.

Mrs. Coleman and her older daughter, Libby, are initially who taught me that I was worth loving and that I could give love in return. When I was old enough, I would wave to my older sister and my cousins across the street while I played alone in the Coleman's front yard. My mom, my aunt, and her husband lived with my grandmother at that time. My maternal grandfather died a year before I was born. My mother lived there because of the divorce from my older sister's father. She also helped out my grandmother financially, since my grandmother was surviving without my grandfather's financial support. My aunt and uncle lived there because he was in the army and had been stationed in England, and had returned to the states without a place to stay.

Mrs. Coleman had a bad heart and she died when I was 5. My security and comfort crumbled. She had represented family and love for me and it was in her home, after she died, that I was molested. How I was put in the compromising position that allowed this to happen to me is almost comical to me now. It just once again showed me how much more important my older sister's wants and wishes were put before mine.

My mom had rented a house two doors down from my grandmother's house. We were all supposed to be doing yard work. My mother wanted one of us to run across the street to the Coleman's house to borrow a hoe for some of the more stubborn weeds in the front yard where she was working. I was in the backyard pulling weeds by hand. My sister was on the front porch talking on the phone. She was initially asked to go, but she said, "I'm on the phone, tell Patsy to go!" I was sent, and this was when I was molested. My mom asked what had taken me so long and I didn't tell her then. He had rewarded me with a fruit pie. I told her that he had trouble finding the hoe, so he gave me a fruit pie. This is when food became my comfort. My sister had no problems expressing herself. He probably would not have attempted to touch her. Once again I ask, I wonder how molesters know who are silent unwilling victims?

When I was told to take the hoe back, I refused. My mother knew it was unusual for me to refuse anything I was told to do. So she stopped everything to find out why. After about an hour's coaxing from her, I told her what had happened. She went down to my grandmother's house and one of my uncles who was still living with my grandma, was sent across the street with the hoe in hand to investigate. He returned saying that Mr. Coleman had denied everything and that was the end of the matter. Nothing else said, nothing else done.

My grandmother had to take me in when Mrs. Coleman died. The difference she made between my older sister and me was appalling. Perfectionism became even more of a necessity for my mental survival. I desperately needed my grandmother's approval. With the A's I brought home, compared to my older sister's D's and F's, I did get an increment of the positive attention I needed so badly.

My mother was one of the most beautiful women in the world to me at the time. I also hopelessly sought her attention. Having gone through the messy divorce with my older sister's father because of my birth, even though he had blatantly had been cheating on her for months (my conception was a mistake to get back at him) she still enjoyed her life and went out quite frequently. This is another fond memory I have of her. I loved to watch her put on her make-up and transform herself from my single working mom into this sexy "party" woman before she left. I'd watch her from the bathroom door, or the bedroom door, and she'd walk by me, once she'd completed her transformation, as if I didn't exist. I don't even think she consciously realized it, but she had been trained by the rest of the family to ignore me in their presence and my older sister was rewarded for mistreating me. My mother and I would secretly have a relationship and in her own way I knew she loved me. She was always secretly my mother. She did the best she could in her uncomfortable situation. However, when she would show me affection of any kind in front of them someone would say, "Why are you hugging that girl?"

I heard the story of my older sister pulling out my baby toe nails told with such fondness for so many years, I didn't realize what an injustice I had been exposed to until I was in my teens. The story of her carrying me by the neck to the back yard screen door, blue from near suffocation from the grip around my neck (the family was out back, I was told that I was about 4 months old and had begun to cry and was not heard) was another story fondly enumerated so many times, I didn't realize the mistreatment allowed by my "big sis" until I was much older. I had a fear of spiders and my sister chased me around the backyard once with a big black spider on a stick, with me yelling for my grandmother's help the entire time. She did not appear until my older sister hit one of the older "T" barred clothes line poles in the backyard dead-on with her forehead while chasing me. My grandmother heard her screams and cries. I was blamed and I was spanked. The next day, she woke up with 2 big black eyes and a swollen forehead 3 times its normal size. I thought, "So God, there is some justice in this world." I had been socialized to believe that my abuse was normal. I have been working on "changing that tape" all of my life. Even within my present immediate family I am still struggling to make myself ***know*** that abusing me is not alright. Any child can be socialized into believing any atrocity is right, especially if they have not been given "a normal model" to compare the situation to in which they exist.

Control of my life became very important to me once I left home. I left to go to a small College in Northern California in a very small town. I had been born and raised in Los Angeles, California. The change in environment was such a blessing. Everything was slower paced and I met a family that taught me how love was supposed to be within the family. Control of my life was easy here. I also found out that not only had I used food to cope, but I've worked to cope also. My family helped me create this coping mechanism also. Since I was so much larger than my dainty older sister, I was used as a work horse. I got all the chores that that a man in the family would normally do. I learned to enjoy them because while I performed my chores I was left alone. It wasn't until I left home that I realized I didn't have so much work to do. I still worked with my comfortable perfection, but not with the fear of the whip. I told myself, "I'm doing this because I want to." Leaving home was the beginning of my saving my life.

I couldn't work after the surgery. I had to convalesce. Perfectionism was out of my control because I had to depend on my family for cooking, cleaning, and all of the little busy work I would do in order to distract my mind from any problem I had to deal with at the time. Any surgery, because of the anesthesia, is known to cause depression. Depression is also another genetic gift I received from my family. Needless to say I was depressed. I couldn't use food for comfort, and I couldn't work to keep my mind off my problems. I felt I could no longer control anything. Every time I changed my clothes I had to look at this huge scar on my stomach from my sternum to my naval. On top of all this, the list of possible side affects I read, as numerous as it was, left out the fact that for the first year, you will vomit quite frequently until you discover which foods your new tummy will tolerate. I discovered this with my first bite of a grilled chicken breast. I thought chicken would be my best choice because it was lower in fat than beef, but the toilet held it down much better than I did.

I have been blessed with a friend, who is a counselor, and he helped me realize how much I had depended on food and work to cope and that I had to find healthier coping mechanisms. Until I could return to work, reading and walking became my favorite past times. The walking helped the weight loss and the recovery. The reading expanded my horizons and my vocabulary, both very beneficial for teaching English. I had to delegate house chores after my sister left, even if they did not satisfy my perfectionist way of getting them done. When I look back on the situation now, my family did quite well, and once I returned to work I did not take some of the chores back. It made life a little easier for me at first. Eventually my perfectionism began to rear its ugly head again and my need to control returned. Gradually, my family returned to the unhealthy, familiar, dysfunction of me over working myself while everyone ***ignored*** my fatigue. My childhood was repeating itself and has been since we had our children. We've been married for 27 years and had our first child after being married for 6 years. My desire to protect and prevent the abuse of my children, and maintain control, caused me to abuse myself with my perfectionism and over work. Revisiting my past to write my experience has been very therapeutic. I've been carrying an unhealthy anger for quite some time now. I realize I've been reliving my need for attention, a reason to exist, and my right to be alive. I now realize I have every right to be alive. I do not, and will not, work myself death to feel that I deserve this right.

The First Year

The first year, the weight loss was effortless. Between walking, working, and throwing up, until I found what foods my body could tolerate, I lost 50 pounds in that first year. Imagine losing 50 pounds and having people say, "Have you lost some weight?" It made me realize just how big I had gotten, 50 pounds gone and people were just noticing I had "lost a little weight". I had to work very hard for this realization not to become another hurdle or road block to my success. Something else happened at the end of that first year. I began to notice that walking wasn't doing the trick anymore. I got on the scale once a week habitually since the surgery and the scale had stopped moving. I had made the food adjustments, I knew what I could eat and I ate 4-6 little meaningful meals a day and I wasn't losing anymore. I tried to tell myself that it was just a plateau, but I knew I needed to exercise. **LIFE STYLE CHANGE WAS EMMINENT!**

Diet and Exercise

I decided right then to start a regular exercise routine at the gym. Exercising at home wasn't working for me because I would allow other things to take priority. We had a membership to a neighborhood gym anyway, so I decided to use it once again. I also began counting calories. That's right, back to dieting and exercising. Bariactric surgeons tell you that after 2 years you have to be very careful because the weight, they say 10 to15 pounds, will return anyway, but you will generally stabilize if you are careful. So I decided to get ahead of the 2 year weight monster. I ate healthy meals, counted my calories, and went to the gym religiously every other day for that next year. As busy as I was, I knew and did not want to do, the traditional "3 reps of this and 4 reps of that," so I did 20 to 60 of the exercises I wanted to do and just concentrated on making them work for me. I would watch the portion of the body I was working and

I would concentrate on the appropriate movement. I finally figured out that all those mirrors at the gym were really put there for a good reason. I had always felt before that they were just put there for the narcissists that went to the gym "to catch" other narcissists.

I still advocate my work-out philosophy. In fact I use it as motivation in 2 ways. I use it as a reward by telling myself, "If you go today, you won't have to go tomorrow," and secondly, I feel better after I exercise. I also gradually added on more weight as I got stronger over a period of months and years, and sat in the dry heat sauna for 10 minutes when I was done because I had read that this tightened skin and was good for detoxifying the body. I started each session with 10 minutes of aerobic exercise on the stair machine (I started on level 2) and slowly added resistance until now, I am very proud to say, I can step a mile in 8 minutes on level 10. I worked with hand weights to strengthen and tighten my arms, and I got on the floor mat to do push-ups and various stomach crunches. As with any exercise program, you should have a check-up with your family doctor to make sure your body and heart can handle the stress. I did and he said, "By all means go for it, just don't over do it!"

Really you are the best judge of what and how much your body can handle and if you do not have this confidence, hire a personal trainer for a couple of sessions just to get started. I couldn't afford that luxury, so I just picked the best from the many exercise videos and books I had collected over the years. Anyway, longevity and commitment to continue is once again, *your responsibility*. I choose to work out alone also. Some people advocate the buddy system, but I couldn't find a dependable buddy. Not even my husband. If he was tired after work he wouldn't go and his work does require physical labor, so he does have a reason to be tired. As a teacher, I get off work at 3 and if I get to the gym before 4 o'clock, I don't have to deal with the getting off from work crowd.

I do have to admit some years ago, before I had my kids, I had a very reliable buddy system with 2 of my friends, but the divorce of one of those friends ended that dependability. It was enjoyable to talk, laugh, and complain about the "pain it took gain" together. I have tried to get together with other friends a few times, but the need to be on time made it stressful. Going alone, I only have to depend on me. I can go when I want and not worry about making someone else late or visa versa. Our gym stays open 24 hours during the week, and one night after grading essays at 10:30 p.m. I went to the gym. A luxury I would not be able to depend upon if I had to depend on someone else.

Not talking also gives me some personal time to think and clear my head. You may feel differently, but I feel I'm my best buddy.

My exercise routine now takes me less than an hour each time. I feel regularity is more important than reps of the exercises you do and my scale proved my theory. I lost another 60 pounds in six months. I don't want to down play the fact that exercising regularly is easy because it is not. When you begin, expect to feel pain and soreness for about 2 weeks. Try "good old" Espom, Masada, or mineral salts baths for the soreness.

Then periodically you will feel great during and after a work-out, and at other times it will be painful during and after again. Truly "gain takes enduring some pain". Not pain to injury and you can tell the difference, but expect to be sore. Expect it, and vow to work through it. You must think in the long term. There is no "instant fix" for a weight problem that has existed for years. You will receive immediate benefits once you have made it past the initial soreness and pain. However, do not expect the unrealistic goals of bulging biceps and ripped abs. After about 2 months, you will have more energy, better stamina, and a better outlook on life in general. It has taken me five years to gain the muscle I have gained. If you begin thinking of your exercise program as a progressive life style change you will have a much better chance of sticking to a program that will allow you to reach the physical changes you desire.

For those of you who are determined to get the weight off without bariactric surgery, you must realize that it takes 1-2 months of dieting to rev up your metabolism to begin you on the road to permanent weight loss. You generally will have this tremendous loss of weight at the beginning of a diet that is mostly water loss. Then you'll hit this plateau that will seem endless. **Don't give up!** I've been there before, before the damage to my thyroid. I was successful numerous times. I just did not keep it off. Be determined to make the diet a permanent life style change. If there is no damage to your metabolic system, **you can do it!** It will just take patience and an incredible amount of determination.

You will also need to increase weight and tension as your work-out becomes easier. If you do not sweat, this is a good indication it is time to increase weight and make your aerobic sessions either longer or harder, by increasing length or tension and weight. This is what I gradually did. After 4 years, I have gotten to a point where I actually "miss my work-out." It has become a part of my life, and remember it takes at least 21 days for any change to become a habit.

Even when I don't miss my work-outs, I still feel the "pain" every once in awhile, but that is how I know my work-out is being effective. I feel great, I have more energy and stamina, and my students enjoy a much more patient teacher. My family even laughs with me a lot more too!

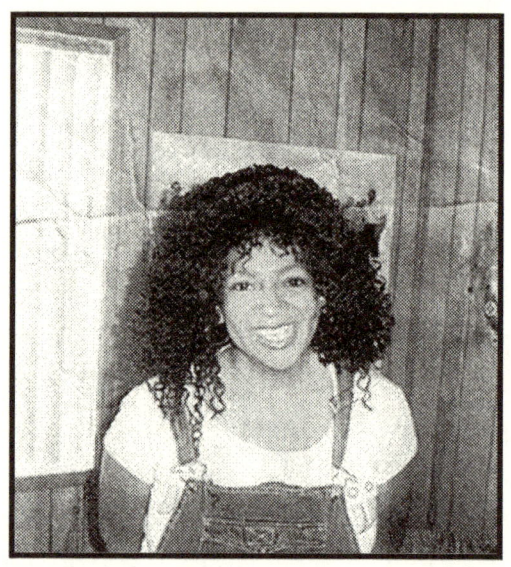

(Total weight loss of 111 pounds. Size 12/14.)

People would say, "Oh! You're looking great! What are you doing?" I would begin to say I had that surgery, their faces would immediately judgmentally drop and they would say, "OH-H-H-H-H" and walk away, before I could tell them I was dieting and exercising also. I started feeling ashamed, that I had decided to have surgery to help gain control of my weight. I allowed other people to make me feel that I had cheated in some way. So I stopped telling anyone that I had the procedure. When anyone would ask that question, I just starting saying, "Dieting and exercising" and those two words put together tend to make people change the subject very quickly! They want to hear, "I've found this Magic Pill." They don't want to hear, "I've had to make a life style change with both diet and exercise."

However, for the first time in my life, (since I was 6) I felt normal. I knew what it felt like to be hungry again. Before the surgery, I ate all the time, ate the wrong foods, and ate for the wrong reasons. Now I eat for nourishment. Now I eat when I'm hungry, and I actually take the time to enjoy what I'm eating. In times past, I could woof down a candy bar and forget that I had eaten it. I felt normal and every one else seemed resentful.

Time became my friend because bariactric surgery hit the news stands with people like Carney Wilson, Rosanne Barr, Randy Jackson from "American Idol", Al Roker, many others in the lime light, and 4 personal friends had bariactric surgery too. Sadly, Carney and Rosanne are struggling with their weight again, and all 4 of my friends have either gained all of their weight back, or lost the initial 50 to 70 pounds and stopped. It is not a "Magic Pill". For me it was a way to gain control and make my diet and exercising a success. A word of precaution; there was a time period between the first and second years that I seemed to loose my appetite all together. I had to make myself eat and take my vitamins. You cannot give into this feeling and just stop eating, thinking it will allow you to lose weight more rapidly. Anorexia and malnutrition are easy to contract during this time period. After feeling out of control concerning your appetite for so long, it becomes very easy to swing to the other extreme. My appetite loss lasted for about 3 to 4 months, and then my appetite returned with a vengeance.

During that time period I began taking over-the-counter appetite suppressants. They proved to be of a great help to me. If you choose to have the surgery, experiment to find which works best for you, but I did find the ones that have ephedra in them made me nervous. I also discovered that after about 2 months of taking one brand, I'd have to stop and take a different brand because the first brand would loose its effectiveness. There are 2 that I now alternate every 2 months, especially the products that claim to be thermogenic and speed the metabolism. You will have to judge what works best for *you*. It is also recommended to have your blood checked every 2 to 3 years to make sure you are absorbing vitamins and minerals properly. Unless there are obvious indications that you are having absorption problems, then you should be tested within the first 2 months after the procedure, if not sooner. Your bariactric doctor will be the best judge, so keep your follow up appointments.

Possible Problems

I did experience some life threatening problems that neither my family doctor nor I can say were attributed to the By-pass surgery. I had an ulcer before the surgery that 2 years after the surgery, bled out 6 units of blood over one night. I woke up throwing up blood and I would faint in an up-right position. My husband called an ambulance and a gastrologist was called to the rescue by my family doctor. The gastrologist cauterized the ulcer and doubled the dosage of the Prilosec I was already taking as a precaution and once again I was told to take it for the rest of my life. Cauterizing fixed the problem and it made me wonder why this had not been done before. This mishap may have been prevented completely and I wouldn't always wonder whether the procedure had caused it or was it just my stressful lifestyle.

Three months after that, a section of my large intestine, right above the rectum, began bleeding. Initially, my gastrologist cauterized the section, and did so almost every 2 months over the next year and a half. The sweet man that he is, even came home from a family get away in the mountains (he was about 2 hours away) to cauterize the section that had be gun bleeding again, and returned to his family when he was done. I had more than18 (I actually lost count) of these procedures during this time period. One night, my doctor was not on call and I had to be treated by a doctor who did not know my history. This doctor asked *me* if I thought the By-pass surgery had created this problem. A pompous nurse, answered for me. She angrily said, "I believe so, we have seen so many patients with gastric changes like this after having this surgery, I have no doubt it caused this!" She tipped the scales at about 250 pounds. I turned to the doctor and said, "I'm not really sure because I had a horrible case of hemorrhoids with both of my pregnancies and I have bled from my rectum before, just not to this extent." Then I boldly turned towards the nurse and said, "You might benefit from the procedure yourself, seeing how much trouble you are having simply breathing and catching your breath when you move. Anyway, how can you be so sure that every bariactric patient experiences this type of bleeding? Besides, I *can* hear you, and I know they must have taught you in nursing school about having some type of bed-side protocol when dealing with patients!" She must have been dealing with her own fears of having the surgery or something, but her reaction was way off the scale. Needless to say I didn't see that nurse for the rest of my hospital stay. This doctor packed the area to slow or stop the bleeding, admitted me to the hospital and my gastrologist came in that morning, cauterized the section again and I went home.

I still never regretted having the surgery, and as I said before, I'm not sure that these problems would not have occurred anyway. That 2 year period was a nightmare for my family and me, but it was a nightmare from which I awoke and still did not regret having the procedure. The emotional and physical normalcy that I gained from the surgery was priceless. Don't get me wrong, I did not want it to cost me my life, but during the healthy times, I was actually living, food was no longer controlling my life.

My gastrologist eventually consulted with a surgeon to remove the section in my intestine that was repeatedly bleeding, but I was once again faced with some very undesirable possible side effects. I could have become incontinent, become dependent on a colostomy bag, or just accept the fact that I would have to stay very near to a toilet for the rest of my life. Neither choice was easy, but the eventuality was if I remained in the condition I was in, I was eventually going to bleed to death. I prayed once again and took the chance. When I woke up from the 5 hour surgery, I felt for the bag, thanked God that I was alive and I didn't have to have the colostomy bag. Then I dealt with the horrible pain for a month. I was in the hospital for a week, and once I got home, I did have to stay very near the toilet because of the urgency. These side effects disappeared and I returned to work 6 weeks after the surgery. I had used up all of my sick leave (teachers get 2 weeks a year in my district) so some of the veteran teachers got together and very generously donated the sick leave I needed. I was, and will always be, grateful for their kindness. I was blessed again. I had that surgery in March of 2004 and I have not had any more bleeding episodes.

Everyone I knew blamed the surgery for my illnesses, and blamed me for consenting to having it done. However, the surgeon showed me a picture of the bleeding area before the surgery and it was filled with varicose veins created by years of straing due to constipation. This condition may have occurred with or without the surgery.

No one really paid attention to how much of my life was spent ill until after the surgery. I was always sick. I've even read that children who were molested or abused as a child have weakened immune systems, and this was definitely true in my case. I was a sickly child that grew into an even sicker adult. As I said before, no one really noticed before. After the surgery, even when I caught a cold or the flu I'd get the negative comments. Some even had the audacity to say, "You brought this on yourself." However, I never heard any one say anything like this when I weighed 315 pounds and had a tonsillectomy (at 23 and suffered with bleeding episodes after that surgery), 2 years of off-and-on bleeding that led to a hysterectomy (I've been on estrogen since 1994 the hysterectomy was done in 1996), and the removal of my gallbladder. I had friends that even had come to take care of me during those periods of convalescence. There was no "You brought this on yourself" when I felt horrible all the time, stayed depressed, and had to take every pill known to mankind and still felt horrible and was forced to function everyday. People just seem to be more comfortable when a fat person stays fat. Besides, I feel I just have a propensity to bleed. If you are contemplating bariactric surgery don't allow my experience to affect *your* decision, but in relating my story I felt I could not leave this out.

I have also gone through the pain of having some plastic surgeries. Something else I have not told anyone about, until now. I just did not want to deal with the scrutiny. It would be ridiculous to say I've lost 170 pounds and did not have to deal with some hanging skin. Once again I was blessed in this area also. For each surgery I had, there were some physical ailments that I was suffering with that allowed the surgeon to fix the ailment, and remove and lift skin at the same time. My insurance kindly foot the bill because one surgery was to fix a hernia, and the other 2 were to remove more fatty tumors. However, I have made further improvements with my regular exercise on the 3 areas where I had the work done. I am very proud to say that my arms are all my own creation and I still have the stretch marks to prove it. My buttocks are also my creation and I have the cellulite on the back of my thighs to prove that, and no amount of diet or exercise seems to remove it. I can deal with these imperfections; in fact I use them as a reminder of the body I have worked so hard to achieve and the body I do not wish to have again. I like this body I have, and I like the "me" I've become.

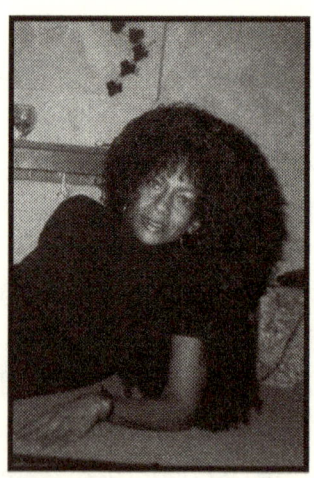

Physical and Emotional
Acceptance

I keep repeating the metaphor of the "Magic Pill" because that is the way everyone seems to view a Gastric By-pass. The bottom line is there is no way to lose weight and keep it off without being aware of what you put in your mouth and engage in a regular exercise program. A person with a weight problem is either gaining or losing weight unless they have reached their goal weight and are actively working to maintain it with exercise and remain conscience of what they eat.

Exercise has become something that is officially mine. I may have to exercise at different times on my exercise days, but I do not allow anything to prevent me from doing so. I have realized that I must take care of myself or I'm no use to my family, my students, or anyone else. I still go through "binge" days when I am extremely stressed, but my stomach won't allow me to eat enough to gain weight as long as I exercise. I do occasionally eat "junk food", a piece of wedding cake, or bag of potato chips, but I don't feel well afterwards and it isn't conducive to my permanent weight loss. I am 5'7" and a quarter inches tall and I am 47 years old, even though conventional weight charts say I should weigh any where from 135 to 145, 145 is just great for me. I fluctuate between 145 to150 pounds, but 155 is my red light to stop, analyze, and diet. Yes, DIET! I am so tired of hearing people say "you shouldn't call it a diet," but I feel if you have to restrict what you eat, and how much you eat, you are on a diet. A diet is a life style change, but it is a diet none the same. I always analyze what has caused me to lose control of what I'm eating with every weight gain. I have accepted the fact that this is a life style change I must accept, and dieting is a part of that change, if I want to remain a size 6/8.

One epiphany I had in one of these periods is that I can not be perfect. Perfectionism for me is self abuse. I can not be a perfect wife, a perfect teacher, a perfect person, and most importantly, a perfect parent. My family is very important to me, but I have got to leave them room to live and learn from their mistakes. Just as I have. I can not be the "Super Woman" I've been. "Super Woman" needed the girth to feel strong enough to carry everyone else's weight. I don't want to ever be over weight again. It can be said that where I used to be a person who would give you the shirt off my back, I have gained the balance to give you my shirt only if I have an extra one to give. My family has not quite adjusted to this change I have made. However, I refuse to do some of the things I used to do, for instance, all of the cooking and housework. Everyone who lives in my home is old enough to take care of themselves. I will still help them when I can, but not to my detriment.

I have gained the strength to say "No!" quite vehemently when I really can't help someone. I've also learned that I can not live in the past. I can learn from past mistakes, but the past cannot be changed. It must be let go, if I'm to move forward. Hanging on to the past even if you have suffered true injustices, just creates anger, bitterness, and hatred for yourself. I was a child who had no control of what happened to me and did the best I could.

I am learning to embrace the present. I use to spend so much time making sure that everything was done perfectly that I was missing joys of the present moments of my life. I'm still working on this though; it is so easy to slip back into that deadly trench.

I'm also learning that true "Forgiveness is Truly Divine," and once it is accomplished, it gives you a peace that excels all thought. I now believe in having hope for the future and that anyone can change. You must first make and embrace the change in yourself, if anyone else is going to accept your change. As I said in the preface, the world, your world, your loved ones are not going to change with your weight loss. You can only change and control who you are and who you will become. I do take a self-inventory to ask what is causing the need to comfort myself with food with any weight gain. It usually takes me about a week figure it out, but I start counting calories right away. I always exercise. I am a continual work in progress. As long as you are really willing to do the work, as long as you are alive, learning and change for the better is possible. A friend told me once that while there is breath, there is hope. No work is easy; some mental work can be quite painful. Physical exercise and dieting is not easy work either, but it takes a combination of all three to obtain permanent weight loss.

I have also accepted the hand full of medications, vitamins, and herbs I must take on a daily basis in order to function. I used to really resent it thinking, "Why me?" I now feel blessed because for the most part I feel pretty good. There are people who do the same and can not function normally. I used to be one of them. I know I must keep this routine, but I can lead a normal life.

I went through one very stressful year, starting with my daughter having a car accident that totaled our family vehicle (it's a blessing she survived), my son moved out, my daughter took ill, 2 of our very close friends committed suicide, and my husband and I almost divorced (just to mention a few of the problems I was dealing with because there were more). During this time period I allowed myself to get to 170 pounds before I came to my senses, but I did catch it. **Yes!** You can eat enough little meals or drink enough shakes to pack on the weight. (Not a Magic Pill!) If food has been used as a comfort, as stated before, you can become very creative in over riding the preventative of the surgery. Besides, each time you eat more than you should, the tummy stretches a little each time. Some have had to go back in for a second surgery because they have allowed themselves to "fill-up" so many times that their new little tummy has become, once again a normal sized stomach. You must stay very aware of yourself. Not to the point of unhealthy selfishness, but be aware that you are important enough to take care of yourself first.

I had saved most of my "thin clothes" in assorted sizes, so I didn't really have to go shopping until I reached my goal weight. It took 3 shopping trips for me to make the emotional adjustment that I was no longer overweight. If the garment came in small, medium, or large, I would unconsciously pick up the large and would have to make the 2 trips back to the rack to get the small. I can finally dress how I want to dress. I actually shock my husband with my taste and choices in attire. Not that they are immodest, but I had become the "large, spandex pants with big shirts" type of person on a daily basis. When I would dress up, it would be a tank-top-dress with some type of coat, jacket, or uniquely designed cover-up to hide the fat. I am a seamstress also and I mentally could not go shopping while I was overweight. I made everything I wore except for the spandex pants.

I have made the adjustment. I am a thin person. I eat like a thin person. I wear a small, I am small, I can fit through turn stiles, and getting dressed to go somewhere is simply a decision of what I want to wear, not what I have to wear. I was never comfortable being overweight, some people are and that is fine for them. This next statement is not meant to offend anyone, but when I was overweight, I found people who would disgust others by wearing clothes that did not cover-up the bumps and bulges simply disgusting. That's why I shocked my husband when I could actually choose what I wanted to wear. I love feminine sophisticated clothing, and I can say with all modesty that I am a beautiful sophisticated woman who can turn heads when I walk into a room. Not just the heads of men either, a woman knows she is looking prê-t-t-t-ty good when other women "give you the twice over to see just what you've got". I am truly not conceited, but I do like how I look.

A New Life

I am living a new life. I can shop where I want. My tummy helps me maintain control when my life gets out of control. I had not realized it before, but my sense of low self-esteem, due to my weight, was unconsciously sensed by my daughter. It wasn't until she was about 12 that I realized it, but she had unconsciously picked up my sense of low self-esteem. We went shopping and she would only pick out clothing that would hide her body. We had a long talk about why mommy wore big shirts and spandex pants, but she was a beautiful person inside and out, and had nothing to hide. At that time she had began to develop a very nice little figure. However, she also unconsciously picked up my misuse of food for comfort. Her weight problem began at about 14. She is 19 now.

I am now an example of someone who truly likes themselves. My daughter is a beautiful person and I have shown her how to feel like a beautiful person inside and out. When my weight loss began, her weight loss began. With the tragedies she has dealt with she had to begin her mental work much earlier than I did. Her weight is slowly coming down. She has already found healthier coping mechanisms. She is an excellent drummer, loves to draw, make videos setting them to music, and talks when she needs to talk. She is also very good at letting you know when she doesn't want to be bothered. I am so thankful that she caught her problem before it became a life long battle. She was the person who made me realize I was ashamed of getting the procedure done. She has been my little errand-running-buddy since she could walk and she is very observant. She has been a witness to almost all of my interactions with other people and she was 18 when she bought this to my attention. One day she asked me, "Mom why are you ashamed of your surgery? You live at the gym and you're always on a diet, you are working very hard to keep the weight off. You should be proud of yourself and share your success with other people." She was part of my inspiration to put my experience in print. The other motivator was having 3 women at my health club ask me to show them my arm work-out routine.

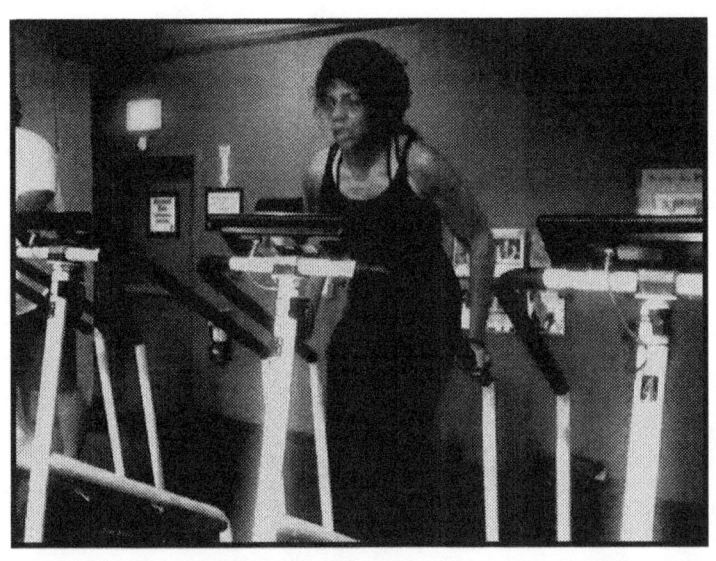

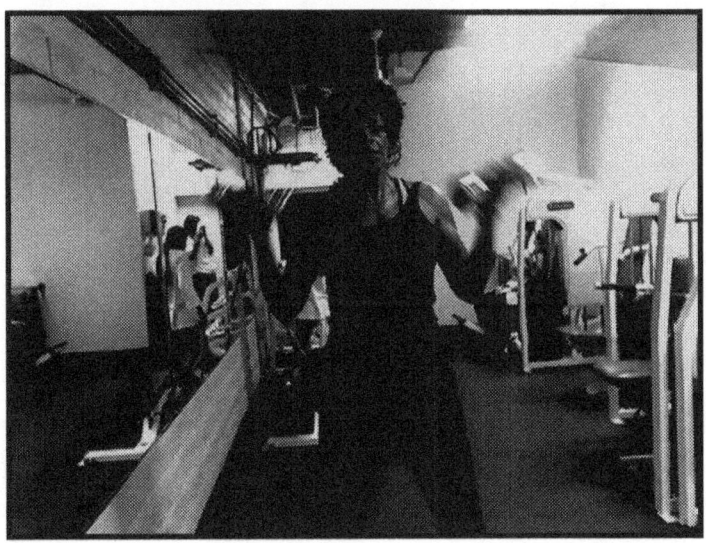

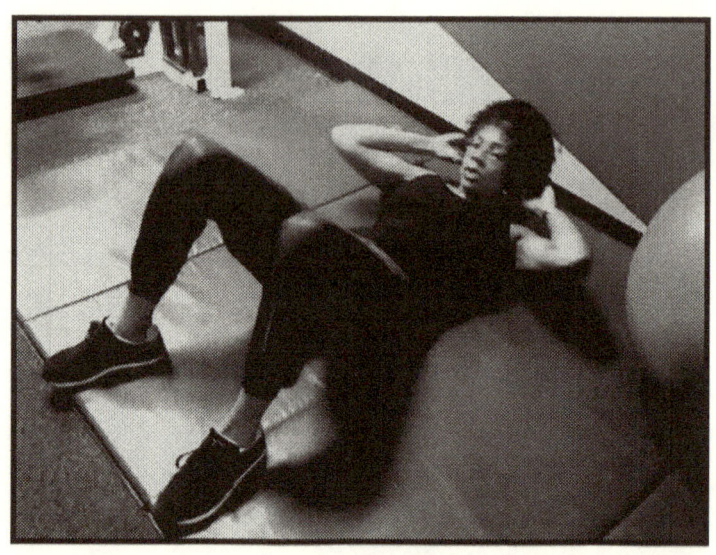

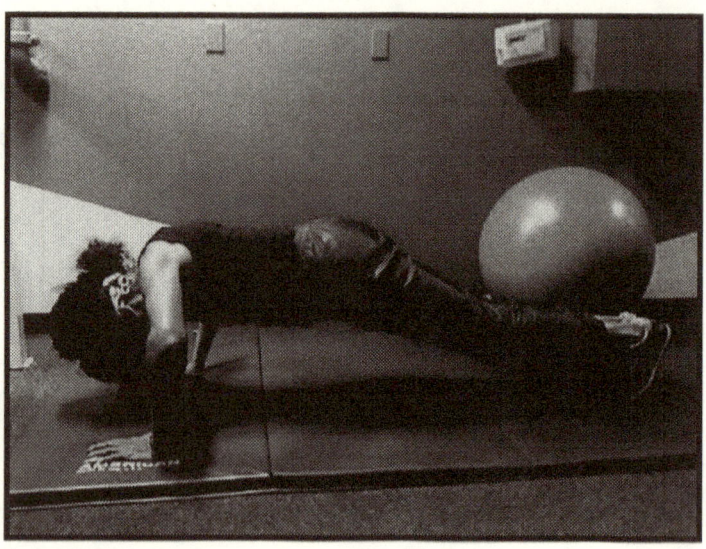

I know I will always have to watch what I eat and exercise to keep the figure I have created. I have learned to treat myself with things other than food. When funds will allow, a pedicure does a lot toward making me feel pampered. A massage does wonders for stress and those unexplained body aches. When I can, a treatment at a day spa is just heavenly, but learn to reward yourself, your body, with rituals that do not depend on food or on other people. This may sound as though this is directed to women, but even you men out there that may feel "pampering" really isn't necessary, you need to find some constructive way to comfort and reward yourself.

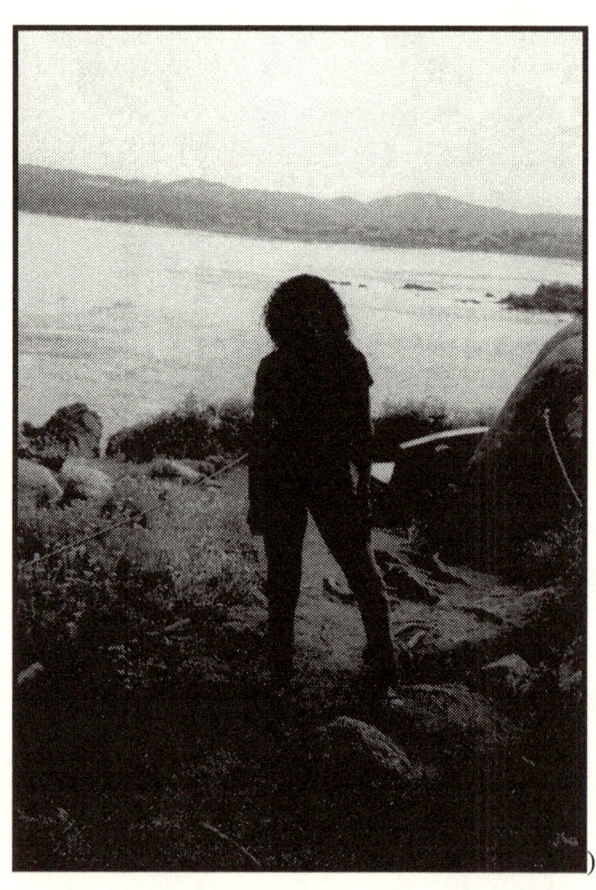

I am not ashamed anymore. The friends, and fat friends, that sit in judgment of me can do so, but I don't care anymore. Maintaining the body I have now takes hard work and dedication. I actually travel, I want to go places, and I like going to gatherings. I want to see the world. I am no longer afraid, or worried about, the world seeing me.

I now know that in order to keep feeling and looking like this…

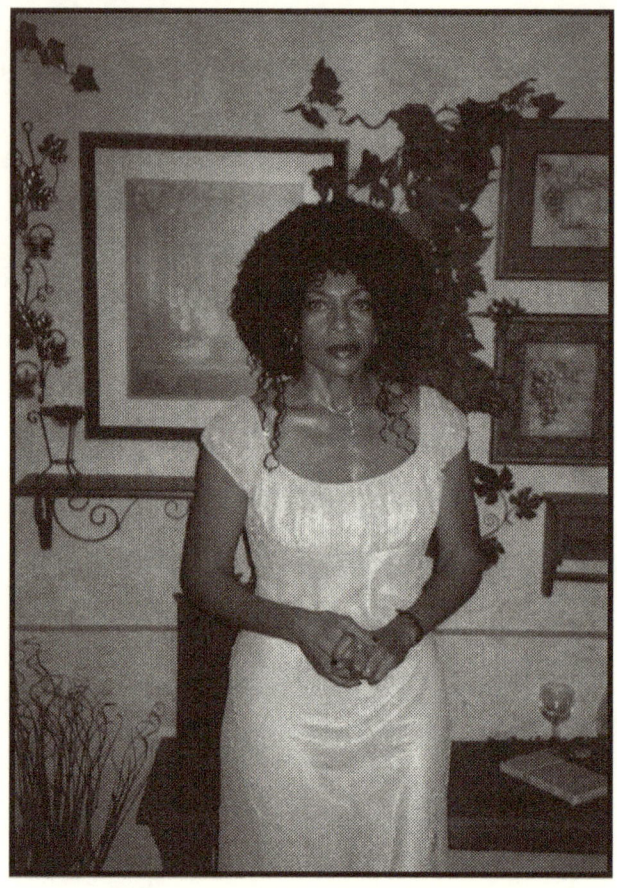

(Total weight loss 170. Size 6/8)

Exercise must be a part of the new life I have created and my Bariactric Surgery helped create this life.

About The Author

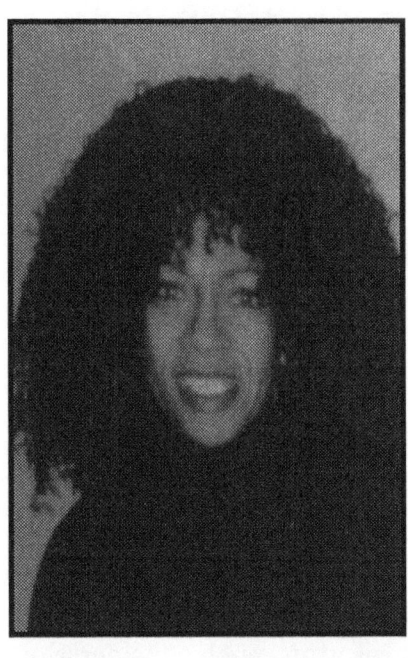

My name is Patsy Winzey, wife, and mother of 2 young-adults. I was born in 1959 in bustling Los Angeles, California. College took me to the small town of Turlock, and I prefer the slower pace of small town life much more than big city life. I deal with the everyday problems of every other working wife and mother. Cleaning, shopping, and maintaining a relationship with my husband, and trying to direct my children in the right direction to help them become happy, self-sufficient, and self-supporting adults. I am an English/History teacher at a Middle school in Delhi, California. I enjoy my students and my life, but the life of a thinner person has made life much more enjoyable. I received my BA from Stanislaus University in Turlock, California. I chose to receive my teaching credential from Chapman University in Modesto, California. This book is my first attempt to have my writing published. However, I did win an essay contest at Stanislaus which awarded me a scholarship that helped defer some of my expenses while I was attending that college. I am 47 years old and have spent most of my life over weight. I've enjoyed the freeness of living within my appropriate weight range for about 4 years. I have had a life long struggle with my weight since the age of 6. I was molested at this age and some of the scars because of that event will always be with me, but realizing that these events were the catalyst for my weight struggle helped me overcome a portion of the battle. After years of life long yo-yo dieting, I also had to realize that metabolic changes had occurred in my body that made permanent weight loss impossible for me. I turned to bariatric surgery after much consideration and mounting health problems, but it did supply a portion of the answer to permanent weight loss.

www.ingramcontent.com/pod-product-compliance
Lightning Source LLC
Chambersburg PA
CBHW021238280526
45784CB00005B/2144